YOUR KNOWLEDGE HAS VALUE

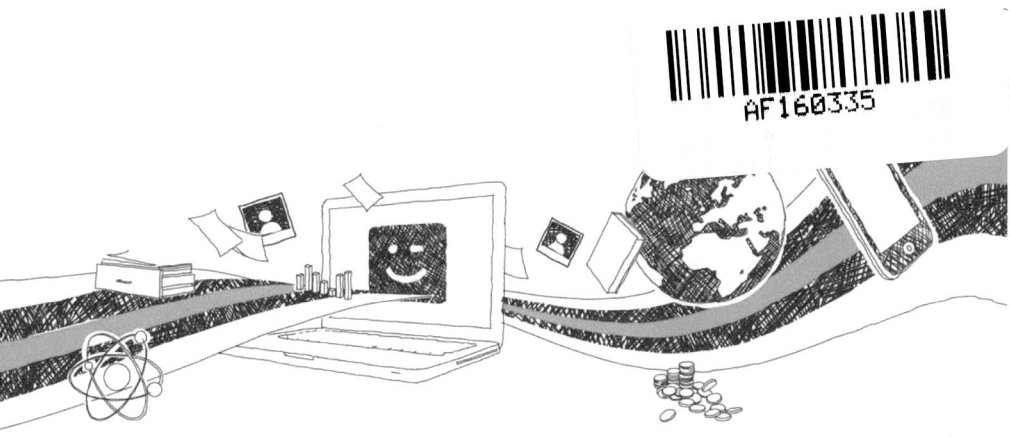

- We will publish your bachelor's and master's thesis, essays and papers

- Your own eBook and book -
  sold worldwide in all relevant shops

- Earn money with each sale

Upload your text at www.GRIN.com
and publish for free

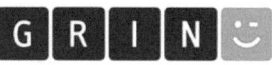

Bibliographic information published by the German National Library:

The German National Library lists this publication in the National Bibliography; detailed bibliographic data are available on the Internet at http://dnb.dnb.de .

This book is copyright material and must not be copied, reproduced, transferred, distributed, leased, licensed or publicly performed or used in any way except as specifically permitted in writing by the publishers, as allowed under the terms and conditions under which it was purchased or as strictly permitted by applicable copyright law. Any unauthorized distribution or use of this text may be a direct infringement of the author s and publisher s rights and those responsible may be liable in law accordingly.

Imprint:

Copyright © 2017 GRIN Verlag, Open Publishing GmbH
Print and binding: Books on Demand GmbH, Norderstedt Germany
ISBN: 9783668581869

This book at GRIN:

http://www.grin.com/en/e-book/380721/social-determinants-of-health-and-well-being-health-inequality-in-the

Patrick Kimuyu

Social Determinants of Health and Well-Being. Health Inequality in the United Kingdom

GRIN Publishing

GRIN - Your knowledge has value

Since its foundation in 1998, GRIN has specialized in publishing academic texts by students, college teachers and other academics as e-book and printed book. The website www.grin.com is an ideal platform for presenting term papers, final papers, scientific essays, dissertations and specialist books.

Visit us on the internet:

http://www.grin.com/

http://www.facebook.com/grincom

http://www.twitter.com/grin_com

SOCIAL DETERMINANTS OF HEALTH AND WELLBEING: EXPLAINING HEALTH

INEQUITIES

Name: Patrick K. Kimuyu

Introduction 2
Overview of Health Inequalities 2
Upstream Medical Model 4
Health Status Inequalities in UK 5
Health Inequity and People with Learning Disabilities 9
References 11

Introduction

Health inequalities appear to be a global, national and a local issue, which has remained potential challenge health and wellbeing of the global population. It has emerged that there has been significant differences in health status of different social groups among the global populations. Currently, there are several health gaps, which are believed to be the principal determinants of the length and quality of life a given individual enjoys. Healthcare reports indicate that some population groups experience improved lifestyles with proper health status, whereas other social groups experience poor health status, owing to their biological or social status. In a community, whereby significant health status gaps exist, the population is divided into blocks on the basis of health status. Health inequalities can be identified depending on different parameters, especially with regard to health. It is worth noting that, life expectancy in developed countries such as the United Kingdom has increased significantly. As a result, all countries have come to realize that health inequalities are virtually unacceptable (Crombie, Elliott, Irvine & Wallace, 2005). Therefore, this research will give an overview on health inequalities among people with learning disabilities, in the United Kingdom.

Overview of Health Inequalities

In the United Kingdom, a number of health inequalities have been identified and, several approaches have been put in place to address the issue. However, it seems some countries in the United Kingdom have not yet made appropriate advancement towards reducing the current health status gaps among their populations. For instance, in England, most NHS Trusts do not seem to have recorded remarkable progress in addressing health inequalities, especially with regard to people with learning disabilities. Healthcare reports indicate that people with learning disabilities are exposed to enormous health challenges, even though most of these challenges are avoidable. Some of the health status gaps are believed to be caused by the failure of NHS trusts to facilitate timely, appropriate and effective access to healthcare for people with learning disabilities. Therefore; the global community refers this to as a contravention to healthcare regulations. Some of the regulations that aim at improving the health status of people with learning disabilities include the Mental Capacity Act 2005, Health and Social Care Act 2008 and the Equity Act 2010. The UN Convention on the Rights of Persons with Disabilities also calls for the improvement of the health status of people with learning disabilities (Allerton, Baines, Emerson & Welch, 2012). W.H.O indicates that access to healthcare services by the disabled is relatively low in developed countries like the UK due to mobility and economic reasons, especially those aged between 18 and 49 years.

Reasons for Lack of Healthcare

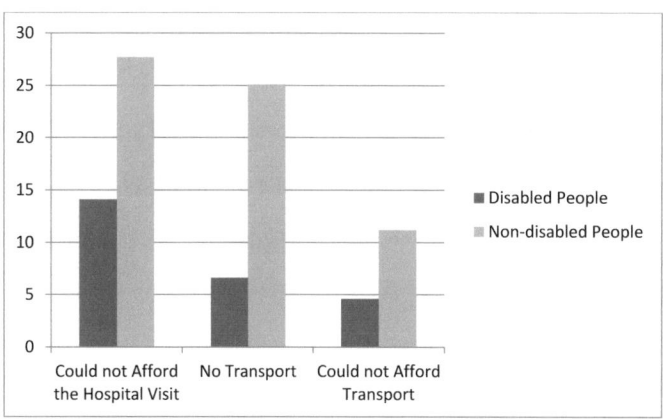

Source: WHO, World Report on Disability (2011)

Historically, people with learning disabilities have always been neglected in the society. Some sociologists trace the long history of experiences of the disabled people in the canonical literature; although the issue is not highlighted extensively (Borsay, 2004). In the canonical history, the disabled are portrayed to as helpless; thus, they have to be taken care of by non-disabled individuals who in most cases do not meet their health and social needs.

Invaluable history on disabled is currently available, owing to the extensive studies on the topic. The three principal approaches: biographical, empirical and the materialist approaches have enabled sociologists to investigate the issue from diverse perspectives but, the latter approach proves to be the most suitable in studying the history of the disabled. In practice, the materialist approach is the most convenient because; it exemplifies the aspect of disability within the society from political, cultural and social perspectives (Borsay, 2004).

Concisely, the history of the disabled dates back to the medieval time, in which people with disabilities were discriminated in the society. In Europe, disabled people were regarded to as sinners at times of upheaval, although they received recognition as members of the society.

Upstream Medical Model

In regard to England, the health status of people with learning disabilities is relatively low, although it has the highest incidence of autism. Demographic reports indicate that 1.2 million, in England comprises of people with learning disabilities, and autism is known to cause 20-33 percent of learning disabilities among this population (Allerton, Baines, Emerson & Welch, 2012).

From a medical research perspective, the health inequalities among people with learning disabilities can be explained extensively by the Upstream Medical Model. The Upstream Medical Models focuses on two principal health outcomes: mortality and morbidity, which are determined a number of health factors. Some of these health factors, which are used as the principal parameters in determining one's health status, are physical environment, clinical care and health behaviours. It also involves social and economic factors as some of the key determinants of the length and quality of life of an individual. In general, people with learning disabilities experience difficulties in accessing quality clinical care, education and employment. They are also exposed to poor environmental quality and, they are not assured community safety. In addition, people with learning disabilities are known to lack proper diet and exercise, which influence their health status significantly (Brower, Egbert & Helmstetter, 2010). It is also worth noting that people with learning disabilities lack adequate family and social support; thus, their mental health is highly compromised. Therefore, the Upstream Medical Model will explain the health inequalities and inequities observed in England effectively.

Health Status Inequalities in UK

Inequalities in health status among the UK population can be explained by the current health status gaps between people with learning disabilities and the normal individuals. Differences in mortality rates, general health status and the incidence rates of diseases between the two social groups provide evidence to health inequalities, in the United Kingdom.

Epidemiological reports reveal that people with learning disabilities experience and increased risk of early death compared to the general population. It has also been found that people with learning disabilities have shorter life expectancy than the general population and, these differences can be attributed to health disparities within the UK population. As a result, mortality rate among people with learning disabilities has always remained relatively high compared to that of the general population.

In regard to general health status, disease incidence rates among disabled people, in the United Kingdom are higher than those of the non-disabled population. Such high mortality rates among people with learning disabilities can be attributed to the increased health risks faced by this population. For instance, disabled children have been found have 2.5 to 4.5 times increased health risks compared to the non-disabled children (Goddard & Smith, 2001).

However, it is worth noting that different health conditions influence mortality trends among people with learning disabilities, in the United Kingdom. Epidemiological reports indicate that different diseases have different incidence rates among people with disabilities.

In general, issues of health inequalities and the disabled in the United Kingdom have been evaluated using the current mortality rates of different diseases and health conditions, which pose significant health risk to the disabled. Some of these diseases include lifestyle-related health conditions, respiratory diseases and dementia. Other factors include physical impairment, injuries and accidents (Marks & Sisirak, 2010). Moreover, health inequalities can be explained by the health gaps manifested in women's health, as well as, the varying trends of incidence of mental health among the UK population.

Lifestyle-related health conditions such as cancer and coronary heart disease seem to cause a significant health risk to people with disability. Epidemiological reports reveal that incidence rates for gastrointestinal cancer among people with disability ranges between 48%-59%, far higher compared to the rate of 25% recorded among the non-disabled population. This is probably so because; clinical blood tests reveal that, a high percentage of people with learning disability are infected with *Helicobacter pylori*, which is believed to be the principal causative agent for gastrointestinal cancer. Therefore, people with disability have been found to record high incidences of stomach cancer, lymphoma and gastric ulcers (Allerton, Baines, Emerson & Welch, 2012). On the other hand, coronary heart disease is currently becoming an immense public healthcare problem because; it has emerged as the leading cause of mortality among people with learning disability. Currently, coronary heart disease accounts for 14%-20% of the total deaths among people with learning disabilities. However, the percentage of deaths caused by coronary heart disease is expected to increase, owing to lifestyle changes and increased longevity among the UK population (Allerton, Baines, Emerson & Welch, 2012).

Respiratory disease serves as another significant health condition which explains health inequalities, in the United Kingdom. Epidemiological records show that, mortality rates among people with learning disabilities are relatively high compared to low mortality rates among the general population. In England, asthma is reported to be one of the common respiratory diseases among adults with learning disabilities. It has been found that, respiratory diseases cause 46%-52% of the total deaths among people with learning disabilities compared to 15%-17% recorded among non-disabled people. The recent research data, which revealed that, more than 50 percent of women with learning disabilities and asthma are in most cases bearing excessive body weights has posed a significant threat to the obese people (Allerton, Baines, Emerson & Welch, 2012).

Moreover, mental health among people with learning disability explains health disparity to a greater extent. For instance, the prevalence rate of dementia among people with learning disability has been found to be 22% compared to 6% among the general population. This high prevalence rate can be attributed to the range of health problems and challenging social behaviours. However, it is worth noting that dementia occurs often among people with learning disability who are 65 years and above and, it is rear among people of young ages.

In regard to mental health and challenging behaviour, the prevalence of psychiatric disorders appears to be relatively high among disabled children. Health records show that 36% of children with learning disability experience psychiatric disorders compared to 8% of non-disabled children. Further health reports indicate that 14% of psychiatric children in Britain have learning disabilities (Emerson & Hatton, 2007). On the other hand, epilepsy and sensory impairment prevalence trends are also significant examples of the current health inequalities, in the United Kingdom. It has been found that, the general population faces a lower risk of experiencing visual impairment compared to people with learning disabilities. Health records show that 15, 000 people among the disabled population are blind; whereas 50, 000 experience visual impairment. Further reports indicate that about 40% of people with learning disabilities have a hearing impairment (Allerton, Baines, Emerson & Welch, 2012).

Dementia and psychiatric disorders among Children in UK

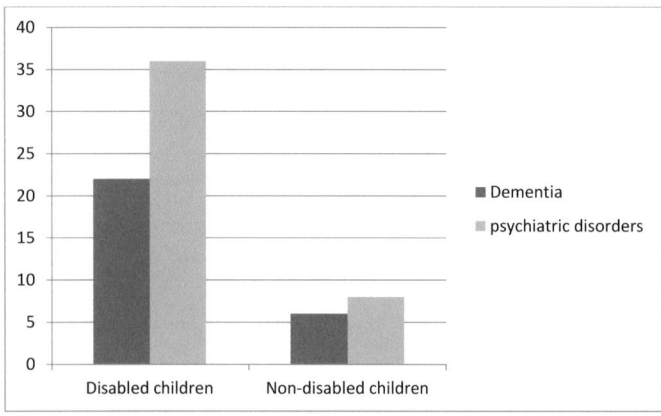

Source: Emerson & Hatton (2007)

On the other hand, people with learning disabilities appear to be facing a significant risk from injuries and falls compared to the general population. These high rates can be attributed to visual and hearing impairment, which are highly prevalent among people with learning disabilities. However, there are other causes of injuries, accidents and falls among people with learning disabilities.

Moreover, gender bias in the UK's healthcare system can be explained by the health status of women with learning disabilities. For instance, most women with learning disabilities have been found to experience enormous problems during their menstrual flow. Some of them experience heavy and painful periods while others experience an array of health challenges, owing to the premenstrual syndrome (McConnell, Mayes & Llewellyn, 2008). Surprisingly, a small percentage of women with learning disabilities receive appropriate medical assistance; unlike women of the general population who are given appropriate medical assistance in the healthcare facilities to eliminate pain.

It has also been found that, women with learning disabilities are not put on the same patterns of contraception with women of the general population and yet they have similar biological needs. Allerton, Baines, Emerson and Welch (2012) remark, "Evidence also suggests that women with learning disabilities are not given sufficient information or are not fully involved in decisions about contraception" (p. 7).

Health Inequity and People with Learning Disabilities

It seems that health equity, in the United Kingdom has not yet been attained because; people with learning disabilities face challenges in accessing healthcare services. However, the UK Government has been making considerable effort to seal the health gaps among different social groups but, people with learning disability do not seem to be considered appropriately because; some healthcare agencies are reluctant to carry out their legal responsibilities (Marks, Sisirak & Heller, 2010). For instance, the Equality Act 2010 requires that all people to receive equal treatment without discrimination on the basis of gender, sex or disability (Mencap, 2010). Surprisingly, people with learning disability continue to be discriminated in the healthcare system because; they are not offered medical coverage under different insurance schemes.

Conclusion

In a brief conclusion, health inequalities, in UK appear to be a significant healthcare issue at the moment. As a result, UK has embarked on various legal approaches to seal health gaps among different social groups. For instance, it designed the Health and Social Care Act

2008 and the Mental Capacity Act 2005 to address health inequalities among the UK population. In addition, UK has so far embarked on International law, especially with regard to health equity to improve the health status of all social groups in the country. Some such treaties include the UN Convention on the Rights of Persons with Disabilities and the Rio Political Declaration on Social Determinants of Health, which aim at sealing the health status gap among different social classes in the society.

UK Government is known to have given health inequalities low priority but, it has changed its approach to address the policy problem. However, there seems to be a number of health inequities, owing to the contravention of legal responsibilities by healthcare agencies within the UK's healthcare system. In general, a cross-Government action appears to be appropriate for addressing health inequalities.

References

Allerton, L., Baines, S., Emerson, E., & Welch, V. (2012). *Health Inequalities & People with Learning Disabilities in the UK: 2012.* Retrieved from http://cdn.basw.co.uk/upload/basw_14846-4.pdf

Blane, D., Exworthy, M., & Marmot, M. (2003). Tackling health inequalities in the united kingdom: the progress and pitfalls of policy. *Health Serv Res*, 38(6), 1905-1922.

Borsay, A. (2004). *Disability and social policy in Britain since 1750: a history of exclusion*, Palgrave, Basingstoke.

Brower, S., Egbert, A., & Helmstetter, C. (2010). *The unequal distribution of health in the Twin Cities.* Retrieved from http://www.wilder.org/Wilder-Research/Publications/Studies/Health%20Inequities%20in%20the%20Twin%20Cities/The%20Unequal%20Distribution%20of%20Health%20in%20the%20Twin%20Cities%202010,%20Full%20Report.pdf

Crombie, I., Elliott, L., Irvine, L., & Wallace, H. (2005). *Closing the health inequalities gap: an international perspective.* Retrieved from http://www.who.int/social_determinants/resources/closing_h_inequalities_gap.pdf

Emerson, E., & Hatton, C. (2007). Mental health of children and adolescents with intellectual disabilities in Britain. *The British Journal of Psychiatry*, 191, 493-499.

Goddard, M., & Smith, P. (2001). Equity of access to healthcare services: theory and evidence from the UK. *Social Science and Medicine*, 53, 1150-59.

Marks, B., & Sisirak, J. (2010). *Age-Related Health Changes for Adults with Developmental Disabilities.* Retrieved from http://ici.umn.edu/products/impact/231/20.html

Marks, B., Sisirak, J., & Heller, T. (2010). *Health matters for people with developmental disabilities: creating a sustainable health promotion program.* Baltimore: Brookes.

McConnell, D., Mayes, R., & Llewellyn, G. (2008). Women with intellectual disability at risk of adverse pregnancy and birth outcomes. *Journal of Intellectual Disability*, 52, 529-35.

Mencap (2010). *Getting it Right Charter.* Retrieved from http://www.mencap.org.uk/sites/default/files/documents/2010-06/charter.pdf

WHO (2011). *World Report on Disability.* Retrieved from http://www.who.int/disabilities/world_report/2011/chapter3.pdf >

YOUR KNOWLEDGE HAS VALUE

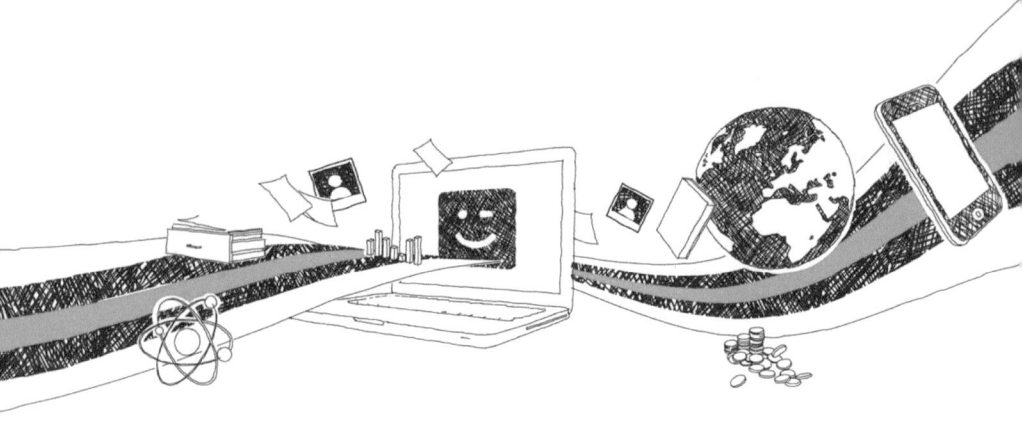

- We will publish your bachelor's and master's thesis, essays and papers

- Your own eBook and book - sold worldwide in all relevant shops

- Earn money with each sale

Upload your text at www.GRIN.com and publish for free

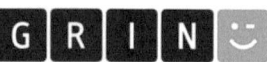